Introduction

In the spring of 2010, forty-one focus group participants met to identify the service needs of individuals fifty and older living with brain disorders in the Fairfax-Falls Church Community. Participants were comprised of adults fifty and older living with brain disorders, care givers of adults fifty and older living with brain disorders, mental health advocates, individuals who work with and/or for programs that serve adults fifty and older living with brain disorders, and academicians who specialize in geriatric services. They called for:

- best practices to promote recovery and community inclusion;
- a holistic, integrated approach to service delivery;
- simplicity in the service system;
- awareness activities and education about service needs of older adults with brain disorders living in our community and resources available for them;
- outreach/cross disability communication and networking opportunities; and
- service expansion and enhancement.

Subcommittee:

C.J. Basik

Mary Ann Beall

Pat Petralia

Judy Ratliff

Patricia Rohrer

Norine Swaminatha

Co-Chairs:

Jessica Burmester

Karen R. Kaiser

BACKGROUND

The Long Term Care Coordinating Council (LTCCC) was chartered in 2002 by the Fairfax County Board of Supervisors (BOS) to provide leadership to assure collaboration in the development of an integrated system which supports the needs of families, caregivers, and service providers; and enables older adults and adults with disabilities to live independently in the community of their choice. The Services for Seniors Committee, one of the four committees of the LTCCC, seeks to increase and strengthen the viability, accessibility and variety of long term care services for seniors in the community.

The Services for Seniors Committee recognized the increase in the need for psychiatric services for older adults and the limited capacity of government to meet the growing need. The Committee established the Services for Older Adults with Mental Illnesses Subcommittee (SoAmI) to serve as a catalyst to promote collaborative partnerships which increase and strengthen the availability of mental health and substance abuse services for adults fifty and older.

The SoAmI Subcommittee was tasked with the following goals:

1. Review existing needs assessments completed within the past five years that identify gaps in mental health and substance abuse services for adults fifty and older.
2. Bring together the stakeholders (representatives of mental health and substance abuse services, caregivers, consumers, advocacy groups and other providers of adult services for those fifty and older) to discuss and learn more about issues at hand.
3. Design and implement service delivery strategies to increase the access to mental health and substance abuse services for adults fifty and older.

METHOLOGY

The SoAmI Subcommittee members searched for needs assessments completed within the past five years that identified gaps in mental health and substance abuse services for adults fifty and older. The Subcommittee did not find documentation of existing needs assessments and determined that the focus group format would be best to accomplish the goal of bringing together stakeholders to discuss and learn more about the issues at hand.

The Subcommittee conducted four focus group sessions to gain insight into the service needs of adults fifty and older living with brain disorders and chemical dependency. Focus group participants included a mix of the following: 1) Adults fifty and older living with brain disorders, 2) care givers of adults fifty and older living with brain disorders, 3) mental health advocates, 4) individuals who work with and/or for programs that serve adults fifty and older living with brain disorders, and 5) academicians who specialize in geriatric services. Participants were asked to provide feedback on the following:

1. What services do adults fifty and older living with brain disorders need to live independently in the community of their choice?
2. What services are available for adults fifty and older living with brain disorders?
3. Please describe model programs and/or services that are currently available to Fairfax County residents fifty and older living with brain disorders.
4. What services are missing for adults fifty and older living with brain disorders?
5. What behavioral health care services are available for adults fifty and older?
6. What behavioral health care services offered to Fairfax County residents fifty and older work well or are services that you would like to see replicated?
7. What behavioral health care services are missing for adults fifty and older?
8. What are the barriers to adults fifty and older accessing mental health and substance abuse services in Fairfax County?
9. How might we build collaboration between providers to ensure better access to behavioral health services?
10. What can we impact in the near future?
11. Are there groups of older adults who are more vulnerable; that may have more difficulty getting their needs met due to their gender, ethnicity, and/or language? What are their special needs and how might they be addressed?
12. Are there other people or groups you believe we should be talking to about the mental health or substance abuse needs of adults fifty and older? If so, how do we contact them?
13. Are there documents, needs assessments, or data that you believe would be helpful to this Project? If so, what are they and where can we get them?

SOAMI FOCUS GROUP DATA

Forty-one individuals participated in the focus groups that were designed to gain insight into the service needs of adults fifty and older living with brain disorders and chemical dependency. The themes that emerged from the focus group sessions include **the need for:**

- best practices to promote recovery and community inclusion;
- a holistic, integrated approach to service delivery;
- simplicity in the service system;
- awareness activities and education about service needs of older adults with brain disorders living in our community and resources available for them;
- outreach/cross disability communication and networking opportunities; and
- service expansion and enhancement.

BRAIN DISORDERS

Several focus group respondents expressed concerns about being careful to not categorize individuals with dementia as having a "psychiatric disorder" and/or a "mental illness." They felt strongly that dementia is not a psychiatric disorder, but rather a physical disorder. In addition, many were concerned about the stigma associated with mental illness and did not want that stigma to interfere with advocacy efforts for people with dementia. Focus group respondents agreed that dementia is a brain disorder and that our focus should be on the service needs of older adults living with brain disorders.

There was a great deal of discussion in the focus group sessions about the service needs of older adults diagnosed with Dementia Disorders and who the providers of dementia services should be. The participants felt that currently, no one agency or county department has responsibility for ensuring that individuals with dementia are served. Often, the Fairfax County Department of Family Services' staff provides case management services and refers to the Community Services Board for psychiatric services when the person is also diagnosed with another Axis I and/or Axis II psychiatric disorder (such as Depression, Schizophrenia, Bipolar Disorder, Post Traumatic Stress Disorder, Borderline Personality Disorder, etc.), and/or there are behavioral issues.

Community Services Board (CSB) staff who participated in the focus group sessions felt that individuals with a primary diagnosis of dementia were not appropriate for CSB services. They agreed that only individuals with a primary diagnosis of dementia who also have significant behavioral problems and/or who are diagnosed with another Axis I and/or Axis II disorder of a functional mental illness were appropriate for CSB admission.

Historically, dementia disorders have been considered organic disorders and emotional disorders (Depression, Schizophrenia, Bipolar Disorder, Post Traumatic Stress Disorder, etc.) have been labeled functional disorders. The Diagnostic and Statistical Manual of Mental Disorders Fourth Edition Text Revision (DSM-IV-TR; American Psychiatric Association, 2000) does not categorize brain disorders as organic or functional (Ameen, Shahul, 2010). Rather, recognizes that brain pathology is the basis for mental disorders. For the purposes of this study the term "brain disorder" refers to all DSM-IV-TR Axis I and Axis II psychiatric disorders.

BARRIERS TO PROVIDING SERVICES

Focus group participants reported the following barriers in regards to providing services to older adults with brain disorders:

- the service system is fragmented
- services are not customer friendly
- there is a lack of resource awareness
- time is wasted in redundant paperwork
- there is a lack of person directed care
- there are multiple providers, but there is a lack of care coordination
- resources are wasted
- there is poor communication between providers
- eligibility requirements are not easy to understand.

BEST PRACTICES TO PROMOTE RECOVERY AND COMMUNITY INCLUSION

Best practices incorporate use of techniques and interventions that are theoretically based and empirically proven to be effective in delivering specific outcomes. When we apply best practices, barriers are eliminated and desired outcomes are achieved with greater efficiency.

Focus group participants called for a "culture change" and a "change in the way we do business." The following best practices were identified as effective in working with older adults with brain disorders:

- PACE (Fairfax County does not have a PACE Program at this time)
- PACT (Fairfax only has a PACT team in South County)
- medical Home
- wrap around services
- community Inclusion
- recovery focus, self-determination
- peer run services
- person centered planning and service delivery
- electronic medical records.

A HOLISITC AND INTEGRATED APPROACH TO SERVICE DELIVERY

Focus group participants felt that older adults with brain disorders often have complex needs and that it is important to coordinate and integrate services better to meet the needs of these individuals. The participants repeatedly recognized separate funding streams as a barrier to integrating services. They recommended:

- eliminating silos and separate funding streams
- changing policies at the national, state and local level
- providing incentives for service integration.

Focus group participants called for:
- integration of Physical and Mental Health
- integration with Medical
- integration with co-morbid medical conditions
- collaboration between psychiatry and other medical disciplines
- connecting medical/psych/substance abuse
- holistic care approach
- consistency in delivery of care

SIMPLICITY

Focus group participants agreed that simplicity was needed in the system. They felt the service system is too fragmented – that it was difficult for those needing assistance to know where to go for help. The CSB provides psychiatric services to older adults including case management, therapy, and medication prescription and monitoring by a psychiatrist. The Fairfax County Division of Adult and Aging Services and the Fairfax Area Agency on Aging provide care management services, caregiver support and respite, in-home services, meals on wheels, volunteer services, and assistance for people needing senior housing.

There is a great deal of overlap in the system and older adults may be working with more than one agency, all providing similar services. Focus group participants recommended the following:

- reduce fragmentation in services
- co-locate services so that older adults can obtain psychiatric and medical treatment and obtain medications at one location
- streamline and simplify paperwork.

AWARENESS AND EDUCATION

Focus group participants felt there was a need for awareness and education activities for individuals, the community at large, service providers, law officers and the medical community in regards to the service needs of older adults with brain disorders living in our community and resources available. Respondents overwhelmingly expressed concern about the lack of formal gerontology education and training in Fairfax County and the Northern Virginia Area. Focus group participants recommended:

Resource Awareness

- a resource map of services available
- information on how to access services
- training on the Fairfax County 211 # - Front door access
- information on Senior Navigator, Network of Care and Disability Navigator.

Education

- education for the Community-at- large
- education on all brain disorders (education on both dementia or cognitive disorders and emotional disorders such as Schizophrenia and Depression)
- education on the impact these illnesses have on the individual and on the family
- education on services that are available and or techniques that may be helpful in working and living with people with brain disorders
- more knowledgeable/trained service providers
- use nurses to provide education
- training for service providers on the whole system of care – few providers have the "big picture"
- education on universal design to promote independence
- education for people on *stages of change* to promote self-efficacy
- education for the medical community on addictions (we need knowledgeable providers and a knowledgeable community)
- need university training for nurses, recreation therapists, etc
- professionals need gerontology components in their training
- we need specialized training in geriatrics for medical doctors after they are out of residency and/or practicing
- Better use of workshops and on-line courses.

OUTREACH AND NETWORKING

Older adults and their families depend on an array of services that extend beyond the health and mental health care systems. Outreach and networking are important to bringing together the elements of a disparate human services system to best serve the complex needs of older adults living with brain disorders and their families.

We need:

Advocacy
- **advocacy** and networking activities in order to raise awareness about older adult mental health issues

Care Management
- care management and coordination
- need a better system for families caring for older adults and older adults with Dementia and other brain disorders
- case management (one stop shop with awareness and training)
- care management (older adults require specialized coordination)
- older adults need help with transitions

Collaboration/Communication
- partnership between the medical community, families, and public mental health agencies to help individuals coming out of hospitals and their families
- a better over-all transfer of information among providers (a major training system itself)

SERVICE EXPANSION AND ENHANCEMENT

Fairfax County is rich with services. However, there is a shortage of services tailored specifically to the needs of older adults. Focus group participants recommended increasing community-based services delivered to people in their homes to help people who have the desire to remain in their homes. They recommended enhancing services that are person centered and family driven.

Focus group participants reported a need for:

Community-Based Treatment
- mental health support services (is only available to people with Medicaid)
- Fairfax-Falls Church Community Services Board, Adult Community Services, Older Adult Team
- medical and dental care
- help obtaining hearing aids
- supportive counseling/advocacy for behavioral change
- language support for non-English speaking
- interpretation services for providers
- care that promotes independence
- support and self-help groups for older adults with mental disorders and their families

Medication

- need prescribers
- need psychiatrists with geriatric experience
- need access to meds
- need better management/oversight (older adults taking a lot of medication and medications that interact)
- education to primary care on Psychiatric meds
- lack of availability
- medication management with psychiatric meds in the home
- need affordable meds
- need providers who know the regulations
- cross training of behavioral health and other providers on meds
- help with medication costs / cheaper meds / or help working with pharmaceutical companies
- when older adults are discharged from the hospital back to their ALF or nursing home, they are expected to get lower dosages of medication. This is a regulation to ensure that they are not chemically restrained or over-medicated. It's a problem because often people relapse and need inpatient care again. Also need ways to record/track these changes in meds in nursing homes.

Outreach

- increase outreach to other social service agencies that connect to seniors
- home care/visits to decrease resistance from people with brain disorders and increase trust

In-Home Support

- assistance in the household
- unless they have a physical disability, older adults do not qualify
- the nature of some psychiatric disorders make day-to-day chores difficult to carry-out, e.g., depressive disorders (sometimes due to an increase in medications)

Family Support

- family care planning
- support groups
- education
- respite

Participants recognized the need to increase practices and enhance existing services to help older adults stay safe and independent as long as possible, like the following:

Prevention/wellness

- programs to maintain or increase mobility (fall prevention)
- education on safe environments/homes to decrease risk of falls

- recreation
- help with transitions through the long-term care continuum
- social outlets and friendships
- physical activity
- advance directives – to make their wishes known
- good nutrition
- regular health screenings – general health, eye, dental
- education on how to age well
- supportive counseling and education for high risk older adults – education about chronic illnesses, problem solving
- support groups for caregivers
- reminiscence or life review programs to prevent depression
- consultation for families and/or caregivers
- outreach to the vulnerable or isolated

Transportation
- need more door-to-door
- lack of safe and affordable transportation
- denial of access (no route available)
- poor quality
- Logisticare (lack of training to work with the elderly, there needs to be more accountability and monitoring of the services provided)
- inconsistent
- safety is a big issue
- to get groceries
- to activities
- to medical appointments
- specialized transportation (door-to-door, wheel chair)
- prompt/reliable/safe for older adults
- escort/support
- hand-held GPS (technology)

Judy, who was eighty-five years of age, suffered from chronic kidney failure and advanced Alzheimer's disease. Judy's daughter arranged for Medicaid transportation five days in advance (as required) to transport her mother to her neurologist appointment. Judy used a wheelchair and needed handicapped accessible transportation. Her transportation to the neurologist was uneventful. However, the driver that came to pick Judy up from her appointment drove a vehicle that was not handicap accessible and could not transport Judy's wheelchair. Judy's daughter called the transportation provider to ask for a handicapped accessible vehicle. The transportation provider told her that it would take two hours to get a handicapped accessible vehicle to Judy. Judy had already waited one hour for the first vehicle.

Financial Resources
- insurance coverage
  - parity issues in insurance
  - equal coverage for mental and physical illnesses
- access to affordable care
- specialists who will accept Medicare and Medicaid
- financial assistance -- help with food, utilities, structural changes to their homes, for e.g. assistance to build a wheelchair ramp

Housing
- assisted living for people with brain disorders
- housing that allows older adults to age in place
- affordable public-private partnerships
- need safe housing for people in recovery
- affordable housing
- housing in safe neighborhoods
- stable housing
- help finding safe housing in accordance with the person's level of functioning and finances
- safe environment
- safe neighborhood
- transportation available
- community they feel comfortable in
- allow person to express their needs and wants
- should be free from abuse/neglect
- adaptability/Accommodations
- housing with support services, for e.g. medication management

Paperwork/Bureaucracy
- inconsistent application/ to receive services
- too much paperwork interferes with providing services.

PROMOTE RECOVERY AND COMMUNITY INCLUSION

"We need a value change."

- o Encourage the use of best practices by county agencies involved in delivering services to older adults living with brain disorders so that older adults have the opportunity to age in place.
- o Utilize Virtual Teams: Virtual team care introduces formality to things that are happening but in a haphazard and unsystematic way… By formalizing the team, chances of improving care are increased significantly
- o Improve transportation so that older adults can be connected to their community
- o Transportation is necessary to go to medical appointments, to attend community activities, and to purchase groceries and other necessities
- o Utilize hand-held GPS technology on specialized transportation
- o Supportive housing: Consult with key stakeholders in housing design. Tenant choice is critical in housing design for seniors. They should be involved in the planning, particularly with respect to design and layout
- o Transition planning: Facilitate individual transition planning/life planning starting as early as age 40 that focuses on all areas of life (financial, education, social, medical).

WORK WITH THE OLDER ADULT HOLISTICALLY

"Working with older adults exemplifies the fact that body and mind are inseparable – problems in one affect the other."

- o Support integrated models of care such as the PACE program
- o Departments of Health, Mental Health and Family Services should develop overlapping outcome goals to ensure collaboration to better meet consumer needs
- o Co-locate services
- o Implement PACT on the north side of the County
- o Provide incentives to integrate services
- o Re-write policies and change legislation that promotes service silos.

DEVELOP A SYSTEMATIC APPROACH

"There needs to be simplicity and transparency in determining eligibility criteria."

- o "We need to develop a systematic approach to working with the aging person"
- o Assign a level of risk to the aging person so that as their function declines, the services adapt to their decline
- o Create a centralized clearing-house for geriatric services in order to reduce fragmentation

o   There are bits and pieces of what needs to be there, but the system is fragmented and difficult for older adults and their families to navigate.

STRENGTHEN EDUCATION FOR BOTH PROFESSIONALS AND THE COMMUNITY

"There is an urgent need among health professions to be educated in best practices concerning working with older adults and their families."

o   Expand university training for nurses, recreation therapists and other aging specialists to include gerontology components to their training
o   Promote geriatric training for medical doctors after they are out of residency and/or practicing
o   Provide education on brain disorders including education on both dementia or cognitive disorders and emotional disorders such as schizophrenia and depression
o   Increase the availability of online courses
o   Provide education on the impact these illnesses have on the individual and their family
o   Provide education on services that are available and/or techniques that may be helpful in working and living with people with brain disorders
o   Make use of media outlets to inform the community about the needs of older adults with brain disorders, impact of these disorders and available services
o   Develop formal gerontology programs at local colleges and universities
o   Employers should provide incentives for employees to take courses in gerontology including subsidizing the cost of courses to ensure competency in working with older adults with brain disorders
o   The County should work collaboratively with other older adult providers to sponsor annual conferences on providing services to older adults with brain disorders
o   Use technology, for e.g. on-line courses offered via Webinars and workshops to make training in geriatrics more accessible.

CREATE COMMUNITY CONVERSATIONS

"We need to take time to plan together."

o   Expand the Family Caregiver Forum
o   Provide more opportunities for information sharing
o   Increase outreach series/partnerships
o   Initiate brown bag meetings for professionals
o   Establish a "think tank" –to better utilize County Resources
o   Increase information sharing
o   Expand community lunches with information (already happens in South County)

BUILD/EXPAND COMMUNITY CAPACITY

"As people age, they often see changes in their vision and reflexes. This makes it difficult for them to continue driving and affects their level of independence."

- Expand the use of technology.
    - for e.g. use of video conferencing equipment to make it more cost effective for multiple parties to meet consistently
- Expand transportation
    - Monitoring of Medicaid transportation providers should be strengthened at the State and local level
    - Need more door-to-door transportation
    - Minimal competency levels should be established for providers who transport older adults with brain disorders.
    - Workshops and/or certification programs should be available in the community for providers to develop these minimal competencies.
    - Technology should be used to enhance transportation services, for e.g. the use of hand-held GPS to help monitor the whereabouts of older adults with brain disorders.
- Promote expansion of the RAFT and PACE programs
- Strengthen case management/service coordination
- Increase long term care options for aging adults with brain disorders who are released from penal institutions
- Make use of virtual teams
    - Work with George Mason University on the development of virtual teams
- Need for more affordable housing with some associated services
    - Need to develop additional housing for individuals younger than 60 who have brain disorders
    - Need more in-home services for older adults with brain disorders
    - Increase the number of local supported housing options for older adults who are deemed not guilty by reason of insanity.

Appendix A

Services Available for Adults Fifty and Older

Living with Brain Disorders

Response

Senior+

- Mental Health Services
- Assists with the transitions

ADHC

Assisted Living

RAFT Program

- 60+/Bridge Program

Home Service Providers

- Many home service providers
- Qualification issues

Adult social program

Transportation

- Metro Access
- Travel training

Special needs trust

Alzheimer's and EDCD waivers

PRS – Psychiatric Rehabilitative Services

- Provides home-based services and day program services

Mental Health Support Services

- Medicaid only
- Homebound can receive MH services if they have Medicaid (needs to be available to those without Medicaid as well)

Peer Support

- Drop in centers – Peer Centers
- Vision – Core of Peers/Volunteers – to provide support

Non-Profit Services

- Shephard Center

Alzheimer's Programs

- Support groups
- Referral services
- Education
- Community links

Elderlink

- Chronic disease management
- Public-private partnership among Inova Health System, the Fairfax Area Agency on Aging, and the Alzheimer's Association of Northern Virginia.

Elder Law Authority

Geriatric physical therapy

- Specialization in Geriatrics for physical therapists at Marymount University

Internet Resources

- Network of Care
- Senior Navigator in State
- Disability Network in Fairfax County

Government Services

- CSB services
- Agency on Aging
- Nutrition – Meals on Wheels, Congregate meal program, Reston interfaith, Ensure Program, MOM's meals, food delivery, e.g., Pea Pod
- Transportation services
- Home-based care information

- Consultation regarding eligibility for Medicare, Part D
- Medicare waivers
- Nursing home waivers
- Liaison with shelters to help people who may need and qualify for assisted living
- Emergency services
- Case management for older adults with mental illness (60+)
- "Work Source" for people in their 50's
- Attorneys who do advocacy/guardianship work for elderly people referred by APS.
- Adult Protective Services – "huge increase in reports for older adults in 2009;" can lead to guardianship action in court (Older adults with Dementia and other mental disorders who re not considered incapacitated – need help with, prevention services, a plan in place prior to decline, assistance for families who cannot make their family members get services and assistance for older adults whose children don't live in the area).
- Self-sufficiency and benefits office in the county
- Fairfax Senior Services center without walls
- Stevenson's Place (CSB ALF)

Private Services

- Wellness Center in Falls Church
    - -Younger older adult / SA

    - -Need more specialized services

- Geriatric psych team at Fairfax

Appendix B

Model Programs and/or Services Currently Available to Fairfax County Residents Fifty and Older Living with Brain Disorders

Response

Care Network for Seniors (Case Management)

RAFT (Regional Older Adult Facilities Mental Health Support Team) provide:

- Intensive geriatric mental health support to partnering Nursing Homes and Assisted Living Facilities
- MH support services – 25 slots
- Beds at Tall Oaks
- Short term care
- Consultation
- Bring people out of the state hospital
- 65 years+
- Help people live in the community
- Bring people back to the community
- Preserve people where they are

Senior+

- Therapeutic Recreation
- Mental Health
- Health

Fairfax Continuum of Care

- Senior center, adult day health care, senior residences, assisted living facilities, nursing homes

Family Caregiver Forum

- South County

CSB Older Adult Team

(case manager goes into the field with psychiatrists to provide services)

- Need more mobile teams

Falls Church Cohousing

- Neighborhood villages
- Case management
- Community members volunteer their time to help their neighbors

Hospice model

- Holistic model
- Hospice philosophy
- Medicare and Medicaid pay for hospice – services aren't fragmented
- Payment is not fragmented - no silo

Program of Assertive Community Treatment (PACT)

- Is in South County only
- Need PACT team services throughout the County

Multicultural Center

Alzheimer's Family Day Program

FASTRAN

Psychiatric Rehabilitation Services (PRS)

- Home-based, psychosocial rehab and day program services (people believe that it only serves up to age 65 because of the vocational focus)

Fairfax Hospital (HELP)

- Admission assistance

Wellness Recovery Action Plan (WRAP)

- Best practice
- Person manages their own care

CEP (within CSB)

ARC (dental care)

Homeless Services at Gartland MHC

Center for Hope

Korean Center

- Heigh Sun Lee

Willow Oaks at Birmingham Green

- Designed for the needs of older adults with mental and physical disorders
- Each individual has their own bedroom – helps to eliminate conflict
- Partnership with housing
- Connects housing and services

Stevenson Place

- An ALF that is owned by the County
- Partnership between the County and Pathways

In-home care – congregate care

Hoarding Task Force (run by the zoning office)

- Work with Family Services

Ombudsman Program

Volunteer Solutions

- Help older adults with transportation

Lincolnia

- Co-location of an adult day health care, Senior+, a senior center, and a senior residential program
- Partnership between CSB and DFS

Meals on Wheels expanding to culturally sensitive food

- Only in Falls Church right now

Attorneys who do advocacy/guardianship

- Work with elderly people referred by APS

REDD Program

Morningside in Charlottesville

- GAP

Person centered care/cultural change/green houses

Integrated nursing model

- Integration of mental health and physical health

Appendix C

Behavioral Health Care Services Available for Adults Fifty

And Older Living with Brain Disorders

Response

Prince William County Hospital Center for Psychiatric and Addiction Treatment (CPAT)

INOVA Loudoun Adult Medical Psychiatric Services (LAMPS)

- Has geriatric psychiatric care

Dominion Hospital

Senior+

CSB Older Adult Team Services for individuals 60+

Provide:

- Psychiatric medication management
- Mental health therapy
- Case management
- Family support
- Group therapy

CSB wellness groups

Women's group in Reston

PACT (South County)

Jewish Social Services Agency provides geriatric services

- Services cost is based on income
- Care coordination
- In-home support services
- Mental health therapy
- There can be issues with transportation

Senior+ serves individuals 55+

- Day program from 10:00am-2:00pm, M-F
- Supportive counseling
- Case management
- Recreation therapy
- Health monitoring

Appendix D

Behavioral Health Care Services Offered to Fairfax County Residents

Fifty and Older Living with Brain Disorders that Work Well or are

Services that Should be Replicated

Response

Senior+ Case Management (care coordination services provided in the senior centers, where older adults are)

Care Network for Seniors

Adult Day Health Care, but with increased case management services

Community Services Board Older Adult Program

Caregiver Consortium

CSB Network of Care

Dr. Dean Storer – geriatric psychiatrist that goes to nursing homes and ALFs.

 CSB family support groups

Senior+ Brain health / cognitive health groups

Public / private partnerships

In-service /training opportunities for mental health therapists

- You-tube trainings
- Teleconferences
- Videoconferences
- Attach CEU's

LAMPS

- Inpatient services

The Department of Psychiatry of the University of Pittsburgh and its affiliate hospital, the Western Psychiatric Institute and Clinic (WPIC) of the University of Pittsburgh Medical Center (UPMC) – model clinic

Expand on the urgent care model

- People don't know where to go for help

Community Sherpa

- Not attached to a funding stream
- "We only deal in crises."

PACT – need on both sides of the County

- Consider having a geriatric PACT team
- Take more of a holistic approach
- PACT works well
- PACT uses a team approach and includes a peer and an M.D.
- Goes to the consumer's home
- Based in the community
- PACT is funded by Medicaid
- Need for those who do not have Medicaid as well

Vision Services

- Specialized for older adults, ethnic
- RAFT - expand the program

Peer programs, Bridge Program, NVMHI (long term hospitalization in the Community when needed)

Appendix E

Groups of Older Adults who are More Vulnerable

Response

Various Ethnic Groups

- Latin or Hispanic populations
- Must increase cross cultural capacity / cultural competence
- Language barriers
- May have biases in regards to receiving mental health services

Individuals with intellectual disabilities

Veterans

Deaf

Gay, Lesbian

Hoarders

Older adults living with mental illnesses who need medical care

Homeless

Older adults with SA and MH (dual diagnosis)

Elderly women

- Need safe housing/safe neighborhoods
- Stigma

Immigrant population / undocumented / illegal

Lack of housing for individuals who are actively using

Hard to get older adults who are using into detox

Appendix F

Services Missing for Adults Fifty and Older Living

With Brain Disorders

Response

Providers with geriatric specialty

- Providers lack a background in geriatrics
- Geriatric care coordination
- Geriatric psychiatrist
- Dental
- Audiology
- Vision
- Medical
- Geropsychologists
- Not accessible, not affordable
- Lack of understanding in emergency room about older adult needs
- Specialized services in addiction
- Need education on dementia
- Inadequate dementia services
- Substance abuse and detox services for older adults

Education/training programs in Northern Virginia

- No geriatric programs (Psychology, SW, counseling, psychiatry and/or internal medicine)
- A lack of education on older adults with mental illnesses especially for staff of ALF's
- Lack of geriatric training for all disciplines
- Workforce development for direct care
- Awareness – Community education
- Education on mental health for recreation center staff in the county and assisted living facilities staff. This training should be required as part of licensing standards for ALFs and nursing homes.

Reimbursement is an issue

- Medicare has low reimbursement

Transportation

- Not enough

- Unreliable
- Safety is an issue
- Inadequate safe transportation

Affordable/Safe Housing

- Needed for those who earn more than $1200, but less than $1800 per month (Assisted Living)
- Need more housing like Willow Oaks at Birmingham Green (designed for the needs of those with mental and physical disorders)
- Waiting list for Willow Oaks of 1+ year

Centralized clearing house for services

Services for older people diagnosed with intellectual disabilities

Work and/or Volunteer opportunities for Older Adults

- Income sources

Exercise programs adapted to the needs of older adults

Reconstitute Families

Intergenerational activities

Primary care physicians for many mentally ill elderly clients

Dental and eye care services

In-Home Services

- "Counseling on Wheels"

ETOH/Drug diagnoses and the impact on medical care

Long term psychiatric hospitalization

Judicial System

- Aging adults released from penal institutions need long-term care (75% are on psychiatric meds)
- Group home care for older adults who are deemed NGRI

Recreation

- Night time and weekend programs

Respite for families

- Caregivers need respite care/"pressure release"

Peer mentoring

Coordination of care for people with Dementia

Housing prioritized for elderly and disabled

Caregiver Services for family members of elderly with mental disorders (dementia and other mental disorders)

- Education/Support

Consumer – Education/Support

Weekend support for consumers and families

- Lack of weekend support contributes to caregivers' burden
- Need more social network

There is a gap in services for the individual with serious mental illness who is not detainable

- There is a lack of family resources
- Agencies roles are not clear (or some agency staff are not willing to do what they are mandated to do/or they stall – e.g. CSB staff and UAIs)
- Collaboration is difficult
- Causes a lot of caregiver strain/frustration

Board Certified Gerontologist with CSB

Training for MH professionals in geriatrics, dementia

- Lack of training resources
- Fairfax immediate area seems to have a gap in educational resources (University training in gerontology, geriatrics, dementia services...)

Appendix G

Behavioral Health Care Services Missing for Adults Fifty and

Older Living with Brain Disorders

Response

There is a lack of consistent and on-going multidisciplinary meetings with mental health providers

- Must meet across departments and disciplines

Lack education on dementia

Day program for older adults with serious mental illnesses and lower level of functioning that doesn't have a vocational focus (for e.g., PRS is primarily vocational and is a good fit for higher functioning)

Mental health services for older adults with dementia

- Lack of care coordination
- Lack of support/education for caregivers

Long term beds for seniors between 55/85

- Divide the young and old senior

Isolation on the weekends

Intergenerational Activities

Integrated services with primary care

Reduce duplication of services/clarify agency roles

There is an increase in the numbers of seniors in the shelters

- They have drug and alcohol issues
- They have trouble accepting and seeking services
- They need increase access to detox
- Increase ease of access
- Decrease stigma / shame
- Increase transportation
- There are good and bad shelters

- We need services for people who are "off the grid" -- homeless and transient Dental/Glasses/Hearing Aids – Covered services

  - Their connection to the world is limited when they don't have these services

Primary Care services

- Medical and psychiatric
- It's difficult to access services

Appendix H

Documents, Needs Assessments, or Data that

Would be Helpful to this Project

Response

2010 census

Commission on Aging (Tina Bluhm and Eileen Dugan)

AARP

Beeman Commission

NOVA Regional Commission

Easter Seals Senior+

"Community Action" – Needs Assessment Study – Grace Starbird

Disability Services Board

Surgeon General's Report

2006 – NY State

- MH and Geriatrics

Older Dominion Partnership

National Association of State Hospitals

#13 Technical Assistance

Office of I.G. / State

- Reports

Ombudsman Reports / Complaints

References

Ameen, Shahu. (2010). Organic Mental Disorders. *Psyplexus.* Retrieved August 29, 2010 from http://www.psyplexus.com/neuropsychiatry/introduction.htm.

American Psychiatric Association. (2000). *Diagnostic and statistical manual of mental disorders* (Revised 4th ed.). Washington, DC: Author.

Ed. Sadavoy, Joel &Leszcz, Molyn. (1987) *Treating the Elderly with Psychotherapy: The Scope for Change in Later Life.* International University Press, Madison, Connecticut.

(n.d.) Improving the Lives of Older Americans. *National Council on Aging.* Retrieved September 3, 2010 from www.ncoa.org/#promoting.

www.ingramcontent.com/pod-product-compliance
Lightning Source LLC
Chambersburg PA
CBHW081238170526
45165CB00009B/3105